A Quick Guide to Breast Implant Illness

Gloria Rose

Table of Contents

Purpose of the Book

I am writing this book to inform you of the possible health effects of having breast implants. At the end of the day, you have the power to make your own choices in life. In this book, it is never my intention to shame, look down upon, or discredit people who have breast implants or whoever plans on getting implants. I myself have adored plastic surgery for many years and I have always believed that people should have the freedom to express themselves. However, I want people to know ALL of the risks that come with making certain changes to their bodies and I also want people to be honest about the negative side effects of getting plastic surgery. Too often, we see plastic surgery glamorized in the media and on the internet but rarely do we see people being educated about the bad side to plastic surgery. Life is precious. I believe that each and every person on this earth has so much to offer, and I want people to be protected from unnecessary pain and sorrow. So when reading this, please know that this book was written by a person who cares, and not a person who is trying to instill fear and paranoia into you. That is not my intention.

CHAPTER 1

What is Breast Implant Illness?

Simply put, breast implant illness is an illness caused by having breast implants. The implants are foreign objects made with substances that are strange and unknown to the body. The body has many adverse reactions in its attempt to rid itself of the implants. Of course, the side effects vary depending on the particular person, but generally, what occurs is the body slowly becomes poisoned by the implants and the victim's quality of life is decreased drastically.

We must use signs and symptoms to diagnose breast implant illness because it often is an "invisible illness" that does not show up in general blood work and physical examinations. Many sufferers are even told that they might be mentally ill or "faking it". Doctors in the branch of environmental sciences can often acknowledge the damage that has been done to the body by the silicone, heavy metals and chemicals.

Many medical professionals do not consider breast implant illness to be an actual illness because recognizing breast implant illness is not good for their business. You must always remember that although many plastic surgeons do care for people, they are BUSINESS-ORIENTED and the main priority of a business is to generate revenue. Each year, millions of women get breast implants so the medical world is in no rush to stop these procedures from happening. That is why it is our job to spread the news and inform as many people as possible.

Recently, the FDA has linked breast implants with a form of cancer. So now they are beginning to feel the pressure to release more information concerning the health effects of breast implants. I am glad people are becoming more aware of the health risks associated with breast implant illness. I hope that eventually, all women will know the truth about how many women have had their lives crippled and torn apart by the sickness (breast implant illness).

CHAPTER 2

What are Breast Implants made of?

Before we dive into the effects of having breast implants, we must first discuss what breast implants are made up of. Knowing exactly what implants are made of will help you understand the core reasons why they are not healthy for our bodies.

Silicone Breast implants are generally made of the following substances:

- Antimony
- Arsenic
- Barium
- Beryllium
- Broline
- Cadmium
- Calcium
- Cesium
- Chromium
- Cobalt
- Copper
- Germanium
- Iron
- Lead
- Magnesium
- Manganese
- Mercury

- Molybdenum
- Nickel
- Phosphorus
- Platinum
- Potassium
- Selenium
- Silver
- Sodium
- Thallium
- Tin
- Titanium
- Vanadium
- Zinc
- Zirconium

Saline Breast Implants are generally made of the following substances:

- Aluminum
- Arsenic
- Barium
- Beryllium
- Cadmium
- Calcium
- Cobalt
- Copper
- Iron
- Lead
- Magnesium
- Manganese
- Molybdenum

- Nickel
- Phosphorus
- Platinum
- Potassium
- Selenium
- Silver
- Sodium
- Thallium
- Tin
- Titanium
- Vanadium
- Zinc

Generally speaking, when you have to choose between what type of breast implant you want, surgeons give you the options of either a saline breast implant or a silicone breast implant. The saline implant has a silicone shell and the internal part of the implant is saline solution. The silicone implant has silicone gel on the inside, and it also has a silicone shell. Many people believe that saline implants are much safer than silicone implants, but that isn't truly the case because both have a silicone shell. Also, saline implants are made with a valve system. Often, the valves are compromised and bacteria can grow inside of the implants, and such bacteria can be released back into the body, leading to autoinfection among other pathologies.

CHAPTER 3

Silicone

Since we now know what breast implants are made of, we know that silicone is not safe, and this unfortunately means that it is very harmful. Silicone is made up of many heavy metals and over forty toxic chemicals that cause imbalances in our bodies. We can no longer listen to the lie that silicone is a natural and biologically inert substance. The heavy metals and toxic substances are what poison the body and lead to many health issues that could even affect our offspring during pregnancy.

Common Signs and Symptoms of Breast implant Illness

Neurological Issues

Having breast implants (both saline and silicone) can unfortunately lead to many neurological issues and cognitive dysfunctions. Neurological issues occur when the toxic substances from breast implants leak into your bloodstream and cause many adverse reactions. The peripheral nerves located deep under the dermis are vulnerable to the toxic substances present in implants.

The most common cognitive dysfunction that occurs is brain fog. Brain fog is a general term for dysfunctions in focus, learning, and memory that can create brief episodes of confusion, disorientation and frustration. Brain fog is one of the most common symptoms of implant illness and many people with implant illness struggle with brain fog on a daily basis.

Metabolic Issues

Metabolic issues can also commonly occur in breast implant illness, and varying symptoms can be seen in patients. Fatigue is the most common metabolic issue in victims of breast implant illness. Fatigue is when you have a lack of physical and mental energy, and it hinders you from completing your daily tasks. People often confuse sleepiness with fatigue; they differ however. Sleepiness is when you lack proper rest, so you are too tired to stay awake and focus on your day. Fatigue can be present even after a full night's rest which eventually results in Chronic Fatigue syndrome.

Digestive & Intestinal Malfunctions

Food intolerance is a common side effect seen in patients suffering from breast implant illness. All of a sudden, foods you have comfortably eaten for years begin to cause you discomfort, and they refuse to digest properly. Some manifestations relating to this includes leaky gut, mal-absorption, and dysbiosis. The biotoxins that are created from the slow leakage of silicon and chemicals negatively affect the digestive system and can lead to leaky gut syndrome.

Compromised Immune System

The heavy metals and toxins in implants can also lead to a compromised immune system and many autoimmune diseases. Fungal, viral, and bacterial infections can also occur. Many women with implant illness report becoming sick easily. This is because their immune system has been compromised due to the heavy metals and chemicals found in breast implants.

Effects that Breast Implants can have on unborn Children

Unfortunately, another one of the saddest effects of breast implant illness is the effect it can possibly have on your children. The heavy metals that are present in breast implants will be transferred to your children, especially when they are being breastfed. Cognitive issues and slow mental development can be a side effect alongside many other issues involving your child's overall wellbeing. It is truly a sad thing for women who want to birth healthy, happy children.

CHAPTER 4

Symptoms of Breast Implant Illness

Lethargy	Dry eyes/skin/hair	Hair loss	Weight fluctuation	Inflammation
Impaired vision	Yeast infections, Candida	Persistent bacterial, viral, fungal infections	Gastrointestinal issues (Gerd, irritable bowel syndrome (IBS), acid reflux, gastritis, leaky gut	Heat/cold intolerance
Fever	Night sweats	Muscle/join	Fever	Night sweats
Sinus Infections	Urinary tract infection (UTI)	Skin rash	Headaches, migraines, ocular migraines	Anxiety/depression/ panic attacks
Insomnia/slee p disturbances	Sudden food intolerance/allerg ies	Heart palpitations , change in normal heart rate, heart pain	Frequent urination	Dehydration with no apparent cause
Slow healing/easy bruising	Brain fog, memory loss	Hypo/hype r thyroid Symptoms	Hypo/hyper adrenal symptoms	Parathyroid problems
Vertigo	Ear ringing	Liver and kidney dysfunction	Gallbladder problems	Toxic shock symptoms

Fibromyalgia symptoms	Symptoms of Lyme disease	Feeling like you are dying/dis-ease	Low libido	Sore and aching shoulder, hip, back, hand, foot joints
Diminished muscle recovery following exercise	General chest discomfort, shortness of breath	Cold and discolored limbs, hands, feet	Numbness/tingling sensation in upper and lower limbs	Swollen and tender lymph nodes in breast area, underarm, throat, neck, groin
Pain and/or burning sensation around implant, underarm	Early menopause, diminishing hormones	Hysterecto my	Metallic taste	Diagnosis of cancer, symptoms of breast implant associated anaplastic large cell (BIA-ALC) Lymphoma
Premature aging	Symptoms of Epstein-Barr virus (EBV)	Throat clearing, cough, difficulty swallowing choking, reflux	Symptoms of autoimmune disease i.e. Raynaud's syndrome, Hashimoto's thyroiditis, rheumatoid arthritis, scleroderma, lupus, Sjogren's syndrome, nonspecific connective tissue disease, multiple sclerosis	

CHAPTER 5

Steps to take to remove Implants and begin Healing

When you have concluded that you have breast implant illness and that you want your implants out, it is now time to take the steps to begin healing your body! Yes you may be suffering now with implant illness, but know that your body can be healed. Below are the steps you should take in healing your body from Breast Implant Illness.

Step one - Stop looking for answers

The first step in healing is to stop going to various health physicians in hopes of finding answers to your health problems. If you have breast implants and you have many symptoms of this disease, please start taking the steps today to remove the breast implants and to heal your body. You are not alone! You don't have to feel like you have some unknown or mysterious illness and that your life will end. You have been through so much already and it is time for the storm to end.

Step two - Finding a Surgeon

The second step is to search for explant surgeons who can perform En Bloc and Capsulectomy procedures. The waiting list for an explant procedure can be long since so many women are discovering that they have breast implant illness. So be sure to do this as soon as you possibly can. Also, know that many physicians do not consider breast implant illness to be a real disease, so have your mind made up that you are going to get the explant procedure regardless of other people's opinions. It's time for you to feel better.

Step Three - Explanting

The third step in ridding yourself of breast implant illness is to totally remove the implants and the capsules that are created around the breast implant. Every person with breast implants has a capsule of flesh around the implant. Capsules are mainly just scar tissue that your body creates because the implants are foreign to your natural body. It is your body's way of isolating what it feels is an invader. The capsules should be removed along with the implants because they can create many health problems if left in your body, and they will not go away on their own. The process of removing breast implants is called "explanting".

When healing breast implant illness, you must have a full capsule removal regardless of whether you have saline breast implants or silicone breast implants. Generally speaking, En Bloc implant removal is recommended for silicone breast implants and all texture of breast implants. A total Capsulectomy is advised for smooth saline breast implants, and it is often used in cases where the En Bloc procedure cannot be done.

When finding a surgeon to remove the breast implants, only get a full capsule removal procedure. That is the best way to ensure that the toxic residue and substances from the implants are no longer in your body, and you can continue on your journey in the healing process.

Step Four- Healing and Detoxification

The fourth and final step is to heal and detoxify your body. After the implants are properly removed, you will find that many of your ailments will quickly begin to disappear! There are many ways you can assist your body in ridding itself of the toxins, chemicals and heavy metals. For the next few months, you must prioritize eating a healthy diet and letting your body heal itself naturally. The human body has five organs that are primarily responsible for the natural detoxification processes. They are: the kidney, colon, lungs, skin and the liver. The way that you can aid your body in naturally detoxifying itself is by eating foods that contain the vital vitamins and nutrients that can help them function to the best of their abilities.

CHAPTER 6

Foods and Supplements to help Detox your Body

This is a quick list of foods that help aid your body in the detoxification process. You can find various ways to implement these foods over time.

- Wheatgrass powder
- Chia seeds
- Grapeseed oil (Healthy alternative for frying food)
- Lemon water
- Seaweed
- Bone broth
- Green tea
- Garlic
- Avocado
- Avocado oil
- Grapefruit
- White Tea
- Turmeric
- Kale
- Almonds
- Vitamin D supplements
- Vitamin B12
- Flaxseeds
- Dark Chocolate
- Eggs
- Goji Berries
- Spirulina

- Coconuts
- Garlic

Foods to avoid while detoxing your body

Added Sugars

When detoxing, it is wise to avoid processed sugars. Processed sugars are found in foods like breakfast cereals, sodas, candy, baked pastries, coffee (that has sugar and cream), low-fat yogurt and many other common food items. It is best to always check the labels of the foods you buy. Processed sugars are very harmful to your body, especially while you are detoxing.

Bad Fats

The bad fats that you should avoid while detoxing are soybean oil, cottonseed oil, and canola oil. These oils are very inflammatory, and inflammation worsens autoimmune diseases. Margarine is also a bad fat that should be avoided as it is full of harmful trans-fat that are known to be bad for your heart. Also, margarine is often created from genetically modified vegetable oils, and it goes through many processes to be created.

Processed foods

Essentially many processed foods should be eliminated from your diet if possible. Try to cook foods from the scratch and to eat wholesome meals. Mainly processed meat like packaged sandwich meat and canned meats should be avoided. Meat that has been salted, cured and canned is processed. Try your best to purchase fresh meat to cook, and when eating out, order food that is not processed. Generally speaking, most major fast-food chains use processed meat so try to avoid eating at fast-food places very often.

CHAPTER 7

Health is Beauty

Your breast size does not define your worth and your beauty as a woman. I know that many women initially got breast implants because they wanted to look and feel more beautiful. Whether your breasts were originally uneven, small, and saggy or you just wanted a different look, it is important that you truly know that your value does not deteriorate when you take out your implants. I feel that most women dealing with implant illness just want to feel better, so the size of their breast and how they look afterwards aren't their primary concerns. But I also know that many women feel insecure if their breasts look a certain way.

Think about all the ways you will gain your life back when you begin to heal. Health and self-love takes priority over vanity. Your beauty is not in your breast alone; beauty is the sum of many parts! You can still dress up and take care of yourself. Besides, you are most beautiful when you feel great, and that beauty radiates from within. Start wearing clothes that compliment your entire body.

If you feel that your spouse or partner will not like how your breast look after explant, do not worry. I am sure they will be glad to see you becoming healthier and more vibrant each and every day.

CHAPTER 8

Implant Illness Experience

In this last chapter, you will be reading a real-life experience from a woman with breast implant illness named Angelica. I'm very grateful to Angelica for sharing her story with me. Angelica is a Youtuber as well, so if you want to hear more about her story, go to her YouTube channel https://www.youtube.com/user/mangie1997

Angelica's Story

I got my breast implants back in 2004 because I had just finished having children and I wanted a more feminine look to my body, because I had often felt that my body was disproportionate. In my mind, I felt that having breast implants would make me look more proportioned and provide the aesthetic that I desired.

Sounds perfect, right? WRONG!!

Three years after getting my implants (2007), I ended up having a complete hysterectomy due to severe Endometriosis! That same year, I also had to have my appendix and gallbladder REMOVED due to unexplained organ failure; I was 30 years old then.

One evening, I was on my nightly jog with my husband and, out of nowhere, I had to stop because something just didn't feel right; difficult to describe, it just felt like my body was going to give out on me, which was just the beginning of my hell.

From the period of 2008-2016, I experienced several, random neurological anomalies - from losing sensation in my legs to serious intermittent body tremors – and, in mid-2017, things REALLY took a turn for the worse!

I had spent the last two years going to countless doctors, specialists, neurologists, gastroenterologists, etc. I spent THOUSANDS of dollars on medical bills just to be told by doctors that they didn't know why I was experiencing the various, detrimental changes in health! Hours of agonizing tests only resulted with me in tears and being told that they would do what they could to keep me comfortable certainly didn't help matters; in fact, I had never felt so helpless in my life.

One day, my husband came across a Facebook page about breast implant illness and was trying to tell me about it, but honestly, I felt so defeated at that point, that I ignored him. A few nights later, I was awake (feeling horrible) and doing some online searching – for what, I couldn't honestly say, but, perhaps a miracle! Well, a miracle is what I found! My husband had joined that Facebook page for me and that night, as I was reading some of the ladies' stories, I felt as if they were writing my story, too. I sat there sobbing uncontrollably for what felt like forever. My initial response after the tears stopped was, "I need to tell my doctors!" BIG MISTAKE!

Suddenly, those same doctors who had looked at me with their sad 'we wish we could do something for you' eyes were now looking at me like I was now insane! And the hits just kept coming; I found out the cost of the explant I desperately NEEDED if I was going to have a chance at reclaiming my health.

So, here I was, almost two years LATER: I was over 90% bedridden due to the relentless symptoms my illness was causing.

I weighed 96 lbs. due to severe food intolerance. I was only able to tolerate certain fruits as long as they were peeled, otherwise, I was unable to digest them, and they would find their way back up.

- Negative for gastroparesis

- Negative for H. Pylori

- Negative for celiac

- PAIN everywhere but especially in joints, neck and ribs.

- Chronic EBV (Epstein bar)

- In a 4-month period, my liver enzymes had doubled.

- High TSH levels

- Chronic chest congestion with a barking type cough!

(PC thought I had CROUP)

- Massive hair loss

- Daily headaches

- Heart Palpitations

- Breathing issues

(Always felt out of breath, even when I was just sitting)

- Chronic fatigue

- ZERO Libido

- BRAIN FOG (getting worse daily)

- Hormone imbalance

(I was not on hormone replacement therapy, yet my estrogen levels were elevated)

The list could go on!

I had not driven in almost two years for fear that I might cause an accident due to the unpredictability of these horrible ever-changing symptoms that I was living with. I could feel myself fading a bit more each day, and I knew that, until I was able to get the toxic bags out of my body, my health would continue to plummet.

I had turned 42 years old in February, however, I felt so much older.

I was on the TV show - FEAR FACTOR – when it was in its second season, and I remember telling my husband how I wanted to be able to say, again, "Fear is NOT a factor for ME!" because I felt as if all I was filled with was fear and that was a very scary feeling! I wanted so badly to be that Angelica again!

CHAPTER 9

After Explant Surgery

It has been just over a month since I had my breast Implants removed! On June 7th, 2019, I had my 15-year-old saline implants (including both capsules) removed by Dr. John Rowley of Chandler, Arizona! The surgery took just over 2 hours and I needed a bit of muscle repair on my left side, but other than that, it went beautifully!

Both implants were still intact with no ruptures, however, they were not full like they were when I had them put in. It was obvious that there was a valve issue, especially in the left implant! None of that mattered to me, though, because they were out and even though I was all drugged up, the very first thing I noticed was that the impending doom I had been feeling for almost 2 years was completely gone!

The first few days after my surgery were mostly spent in bed because I had drains and they were extremely uncomfortable! On day 4, post-surgery, I had my drains removed, and oh my lord, it instantly felt like I was free! My plastic surgeon said he was very impressed with how quickly my body was healing and detoxing! Day 5 post-op was by far the most emotional since the removal. On this day, I had a scheduled appointment with my primary care physician to go over how my surgery went! (Mind you, she did not believe that my implants could be causing all of my health issues, but that being said, she also agreed that having them removed couldn't hurt either!)

Needless to say, she was speechless! She started bawling and we both just sat there and cried for like 10 minutes! She then proceeded to call and leave a message with the two specialists from the mayo clinic that were also working on my case; she told them that she witnessed a medical miracle! Then she sent me for blood work, which I was so excited for - that was a first for me! (I had my blood drawn every few months for 2 years straight and every time I would dread hearing the results! Not this time: I was so excited to see where all my levels were!)

For me, the best day was when my doctor called me to tell me that she could not believe what she is reading. All my blood work came back either perfect or almost perfect! My EBV and vitamin D was still a bit wonky, but nothing like it two weeks prior! My liver enzymes (which had been dangerously elevated) along with my kidney functions, were back to normal. She even said that she had the tests run twice because she couldn't believe the results! For almost two years, I had to use a cane in order to walk, and now I can stand on one leg with almost perfect balance! The things that are still a bit of an issue are the food intolerances! I am unable to tolerate gluten, dairy or meat, but I am ok with that because I am finally able to eat again! I went into my surgery weighing about 90 lbs. and I now weigh 103 lbs. and I look amazing! I truly have been given a second chance and I plan on living life to the fullest!

www.ingramcontent.com/pod-product-compliance
Lightning Source LLC
Chambersburg PA
CBHW031922270726
48655CB00007BA/3189